I Am A Yogi Animal

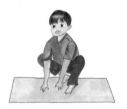 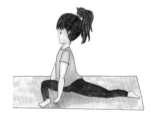 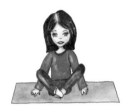

By: Maureen Mohr Bivens

Illustrations By: Dorothy Mohr McCaleb

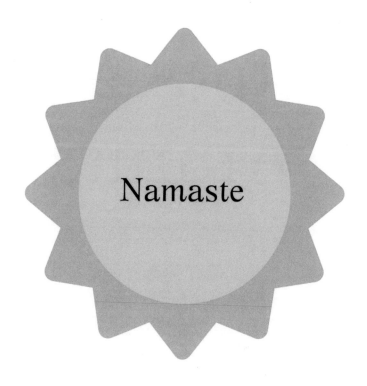

Namaste

Dedicated to Blaise, Crosley, and Basile.

Proceeds shared with Project Yoga in support of at-risk communities.

I am a **yogi animal**....
So strong and yet so kind.
With heart and soul, I take a breath, as peace flows through my mind

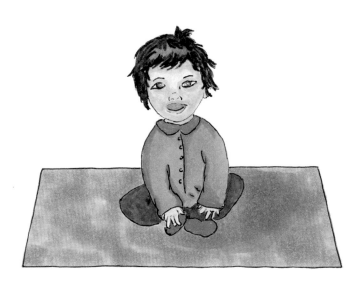

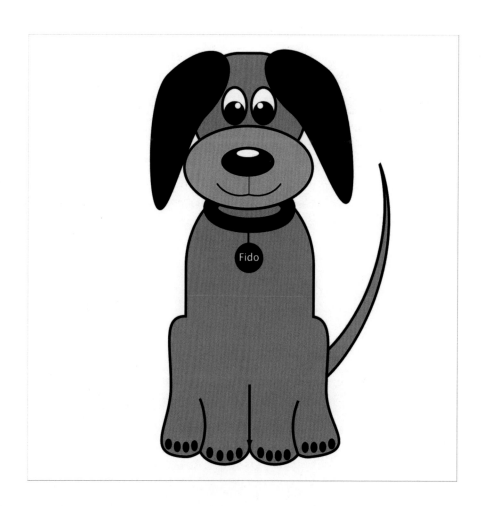

Sometimes the sound of thunder can make me feel afraid.
I settle into **downward dog** and sounds begin to fade.

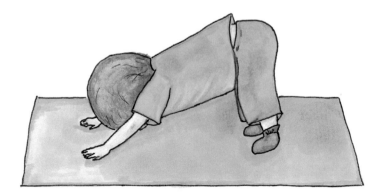

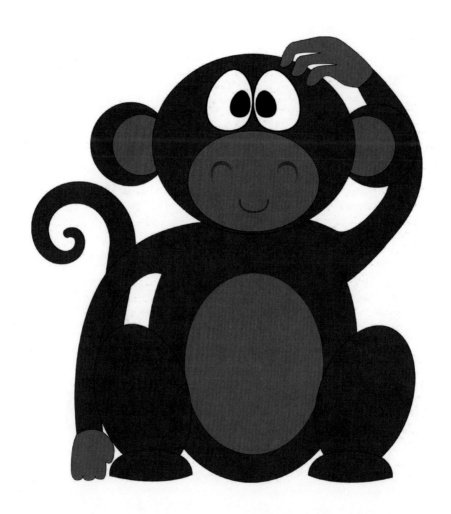

The cries my baby sister makes can often bother me.
But when she sees my **monkey** face, her tears no longer be.

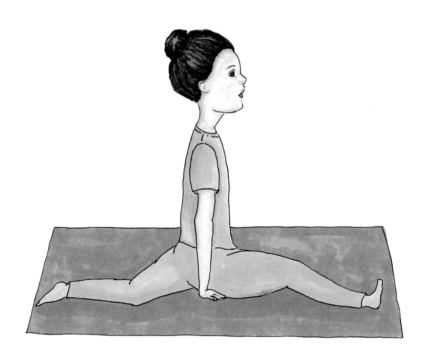

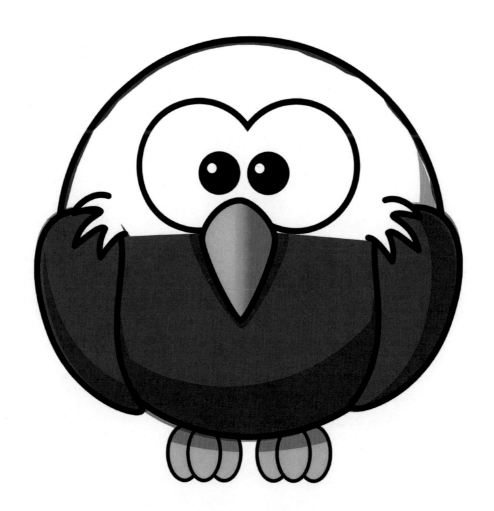

On days when I feel lonely, and often wonder why,
I wrap my **eagle** wings around and feel prepared to fly.

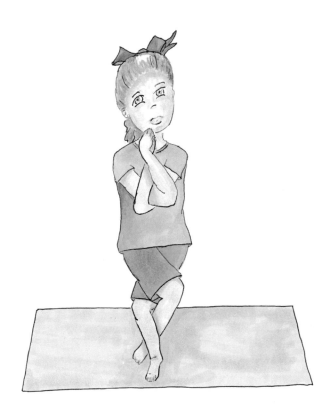

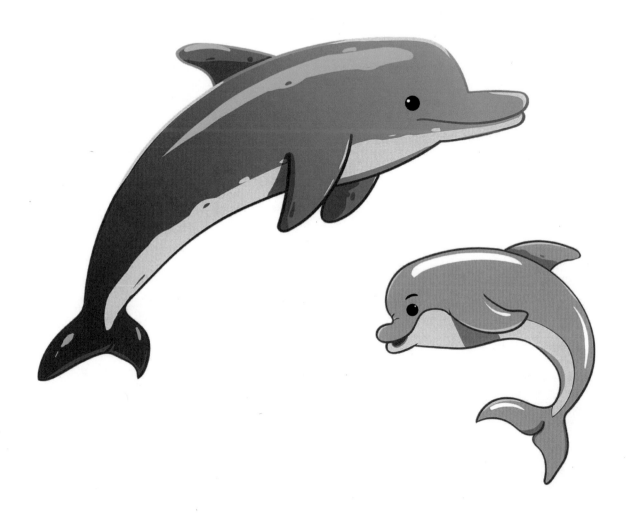

When loud and scary noises make me feel uptight,
I float into my **dolphin** pose and everything feels right.

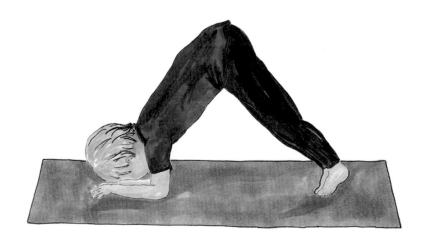

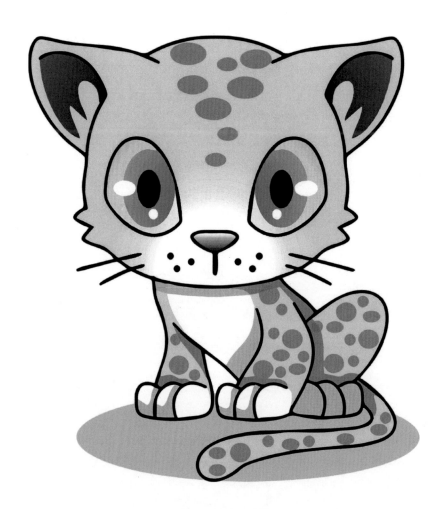

One day I thought I lost my **cat** and didn't know where to look.
I arched my back and tucked my chin and saw her by the brook.

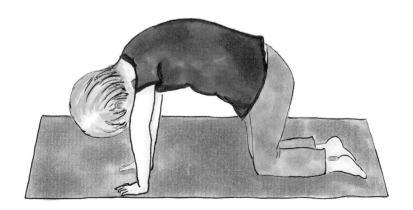

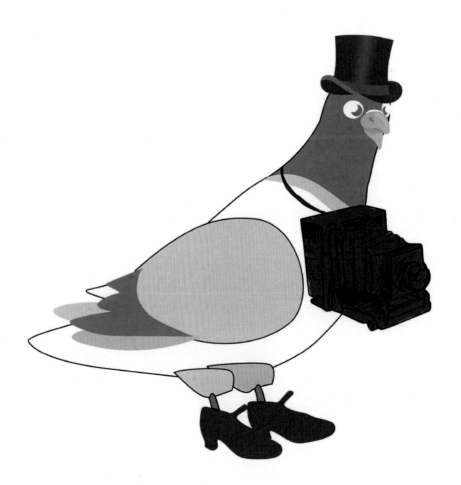

I missed my Dad at daycare, and sat quietly on the floor.
Then like a **flying pigeon**, he soon flew through the door.

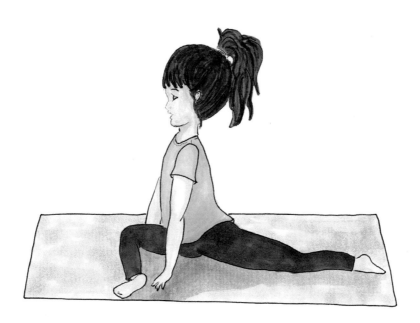

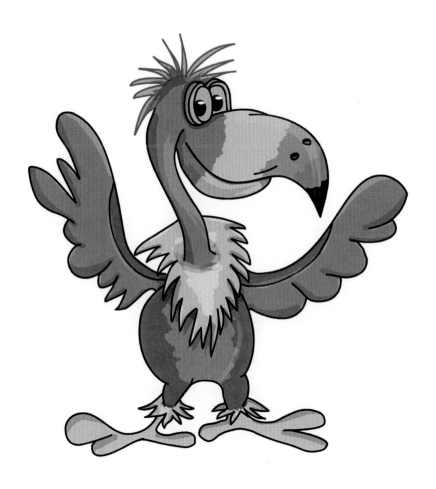

The rain just kept on coming and the sun seemed far away.
So like a **crow**, I swooped down low and found a place to play.

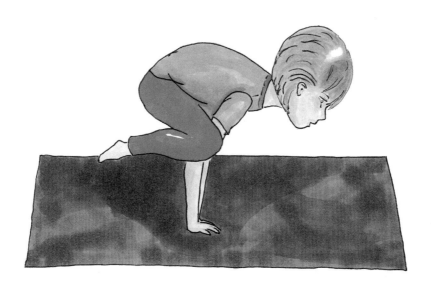

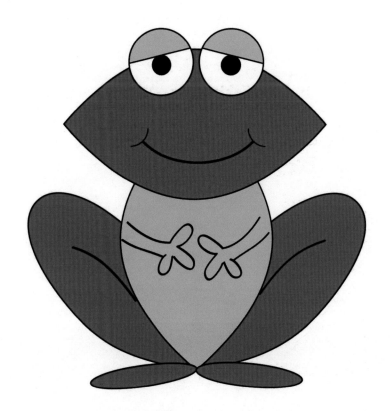

My mama had to leave again to take another trip.
But that's okay, she works so hard, so like a **frog**, I skip.

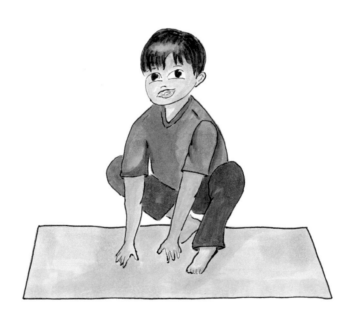

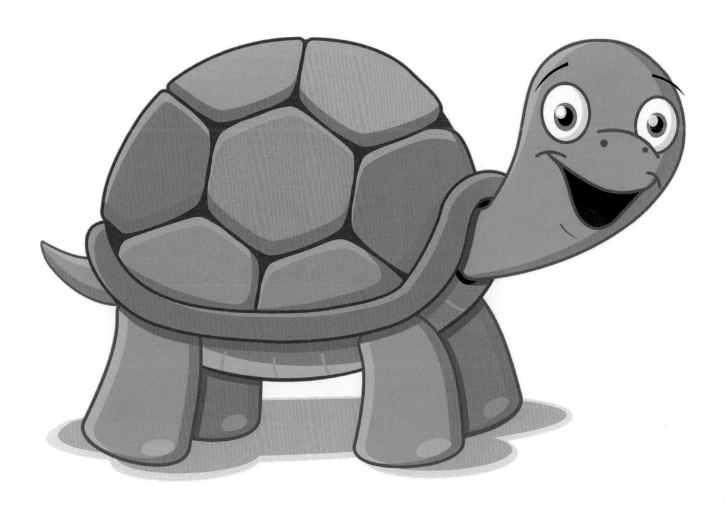

I had a pet named Turtle that never left my side.
So sometimes in my **turtle pose**, I honor him with pride.

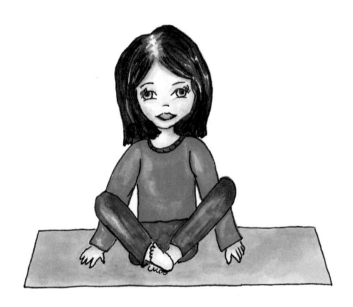

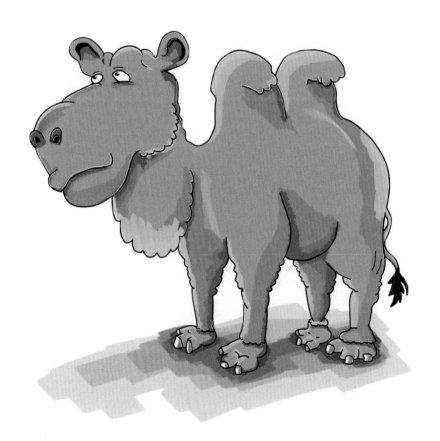

At night when darkness starts to fall, my heart begins to pound.
Then I imagine **camel pose**, and let my breath calm down.

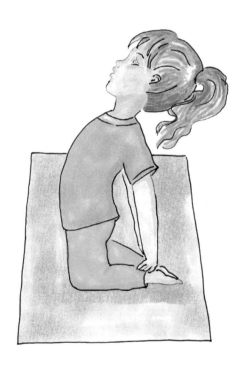

I am a **yogi animal**....
So strong and yet so kind.
With heart and soul, I take a breath, as peace flows through my mind.

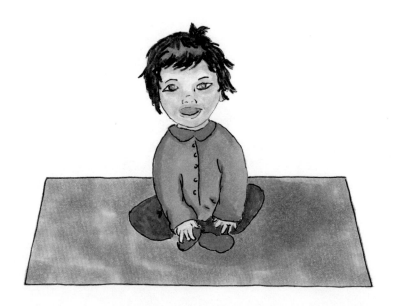

Namaste.

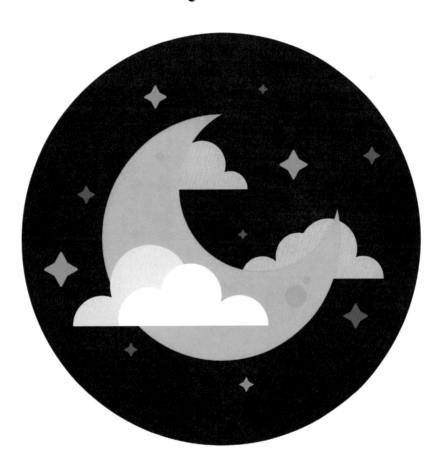

Made in the USA
Lexington, KY
01 September 2018